Making Sense of Pain After Knee Replacement

Why Your Knee Still Hurts, Feels Tight, and Changes from Day to Day

Michelle Losurdo, PT, DPT, OCS
Board-Certified Clinical Specialist in Orthopaedic Physical Therapy

Creator and Host of the Total Knee Success Podcast™

Published by: Pale Blue Press LLC
ISBN: 978-0-9963877-3-6
Paperback Edition
Printed in the United States of America.

IMPORTANT DISCLAIMER

This book is intended for educational and informational purposes only.

It is not medical advice, diagnosis, or treatment and should not be relied upon as a substitute for personal medical care from qualified healthcare professionals. The information presented reflects general educational principles related to knee replacement rehabilitation and pain after surgery. Individual experiences, symptoms, medical histories, and rehabilitation responses can vary significantly.

The information in this book reflects current research and clinical understanding at the time of publication, though recommendations and medical knowledge may evolve over time.

Readers should consult their physicians, physical therapists, or other qualified healthcare providers regarding their individual situation and before making decisions related to medical care, activity, exercise, medications, or treatment.

The author and publisher disclaim responsibility for any adverse effects or consequences resulting directly or indirectly from the use of the information contained in this book.

If you experience worsening symptoms, increasing redness, warmth, drainage, fever, chest pain, sudden shortness of breath, or other urgent medical concerns, seek immediate medical attention.

Table of Contents

Introduction	7
Overview	9
When Pain May Signal Something More Serious	11
How Pain Commonly Shows Up After Knee Replacement	13
Surgical Pain	17
Movement Pain	20
Overload Pain	22
Sensitivity Pain	24
Which Pain Pattern Fits What You're Feeling?	27
Matching Strategies to the Pain Pattern	29
What Else Can Help?	47
When a Strategy Helps One Day and Not the Next	57
When You Need More Help Sorting Out the Pain	59
Decreased Pain Is Not the Only Sign of Progress	61
Common Traps That Make Pain Harder to Understand	63
Quick Reference: What Am I Feeling?	73
Quick Reference: Pain Patterns	77
Final Thoughts	79
Continue Learning with Total Knee Success	81
About the Author	83
References	85

Introduction

Pain after knee replacement can make you question everything. Your knee feels okay at breakfast, then swollen and tight by dinner. The first few steps after standing up from sitting hurt, but the pain eases once you get moving. A trip to the store goes well, yet two hours later your knee is throbbing. You start wondering: Which version of my knee am I supposed to believe?

John asks the same thing. He is 74, retired, active, and spent much of his career in management, so he is used to solving problems. He recently had a knee replacement and is working through the early phases after surgery. Before surgery, he had great success planning and following through on almost everything he did personally and professionally. Now he follows the plan, and his knee still changes from one hour to the next. It doesn't make sense to him. He feels like his pain is controlling him, and he resents it.

John is fictional, but his experiences come from the kinds of things people describe every day after knee replacement.

On Monday, standing up from the breakfast table hurts enough that John grabs the chair. Ten steps later, it eases. On Tuesday, he feels pretty good and runs an extra errand. That evening, his knee is swollen and hard to bend. On Friday, his usual mid-morning walk feels much worse after a miserable night of sleep. Three painful experiences, three different stories.

If you have had days like these, it may be easy to think that something is wrong, you're imagining it, or you're just not tough enough. But that's often not the case. Many people experience these types of situations after knee replacement.

Imagine if it were different, if you could pay attention, choose your response, and start to feel better. You might not be missing the signals. You might be missing a way to sort them out.

A pain number cannot tell you when the pain started, what brought it on, or what happened afterward.

This book will teach you a simple way to work through pain questions. You will learn four common pain patterns, how each one tends to behave, and which responses often fit each pattern. You will also learn when a pattern seems familiar and when you should consider reaching out to your surgeon, physical therapist, or other healthcare professional instead.

Overview

Here is the problem: pain after knee replacement is often treated as one big category. It hurts, so the only question becomes, "How much?" or "What number is your pain on a scale of zero to ten?"

But if your knee hurts on the first step in the morning, it tells a different story than if it swells several hours after a busy afternoon. That's why I often say to my patients, "Tell me about it." I'm looking for the nature of their symptoms and what activities they participated in. And that's exactly what they tell me.

Over the years, I have learned that people are excellent at talking about what they do and how much they hurt, but often not so great at seeing the cause-and-effect behind the pain they just described. At least not until they say it out loud and listen to themselves. That's not surprising, for many reasons, including the fact that they are in pain and often exhausted by it!

So, let's break it down.

This book uses four simple pain patterns to help you connect what you feel with when it happens and which responses may fit.

These patterns help you recognize what may be driving a familiar pain experience. They cannot identify one exact tissue or rule out a medical problem.

The warning-sign section explains when to stop sorting patterns and seek medical care. Always remember that I don't know you, and I'm not your therapist, so this book is informational. You need to work with your own care team for your situation.

Let's get started.

When Pain May Signal Something More Serious

Pain can change for many reasons after knee replacement, including swelling, movement, total activity, and sensitivity. Some changes need medical evaluation, especially when symptoms are new, distinctly different from your usual experience, worsening, or accompanied by other warning signs.

Contact a healthcare professional promptly if redness or warmth around the incision increases, drainage appears, you develop a fever, or pain continues to worsen instead of returning to your recent level.

New or worsening calf pain, swelling, warmth, or tenderness can indicate a blood clot or deep vein thrombosis and require immediate medical care. Symptoms cannot confirm or rule out a deep vein thrombosis. Sudden shortness of breath, chest discomfort, lightheadedness, or fainting can occur with a pulmonary embolism and require immediate medical care.

Seek medical guidance when a fall or injury causes an increase in pain or swelling, a new loss of knee movement, or new difficulty putting weight on your leg.

Pain that continues or worsens later after surgery and no longer behaves like your usual symptoms may need evaluation for a less common problem involving the joint, nearby tissues, or implant.

You might find it useful to ask three questions when you are unsure:

1. Is this distinctly different from my recent experience?
2. Is it continuing to worsen?
3. Did another concerning symptom appear with it?

A yes means it is time to move from the everyday pain-pattern framework to guidance from your surgeon or another qualified healthcare professional. If you are unsure, reach out for that guidance.

For a nonurgent but unfamiliar change, describe when it began, what changed, and which other symptoms are present when you contact your surgeon, physical therapist, or other healthcare professional. A medical emergency requires immediate care.

The four pain patterns help you recognize familiar experiences. New, severe, or worsening symptoms get medical attention first.

How Pain Commonly Shows Up After Knee Replacement

Let's start with four ways pain commonly behaves after knee replacement. This framework is not a formal research classification, but it reflects well-established principles from pain science along with consistent clinical observations and patient reports after knee replacement.

You may recognize one immediately. You might also recognize yourself in all four, depending on the day. Identifying those patterns can make it easier to interpret what you are feeling.

Surgical pain is connected to the physical effects of surgery. It often includes swelling, warmth, pressure, heaviness, incision soreness, knee stiffness, and a band-like feeling around the front of your knee. It is usually more noticeable early after surgery, although no single date tells everyone when it should be gone.

Movement pain appears during a particular movement. It usually has a recognizable trigger and may appear when you bend, straighten, stand, walk, climb stairs, or take the first few steps after sitting. The important clue is that the pain starts with the movement and may change as you continue moving.

Overload pain often has a delay. It arrives later after the total activity was more than your knee was ready for. You may feel fine during exercise, errands, cooking, or a family visit. Later that evening or the next morning, your knee has more swelling, knee stiffness, soreness, or you have difficulty moving it. Your total activity in the day is often more important than one activity.

Sensitivity pain can feel baffling. It often feels stronger or more irritating than the activity alone would suggest. The same pajama leg material that has been touching your leg for the past few nights suddenly feels irritating. The sheet brushing on your knee keeps you awake. A familiar movement hurts much more after poor sleep or a particularly stressful day. The pain is real, but the amount of activity does not fully explain its intensity.

You don't need to choose one perfect label. The purpose is to find the pattern that best fits what is happening right now so you can choose a useful response.

The evidence supports this kind of flexible thinking, and you can be flexible too. Pain, swelling, function, lasting soreness, range of motion, and your overall response all provide information. One painful moment does not get to decide how your day goes or the whole plan for your pain for the rest of your life. You get to choose your response.

I think that's worth repeating.

You get to choose your response.

John finally sees the difference during one ordinary week. His knee is swollen and sore early in the week. Maybe he is experiencing surgical pain. Standing up brings a pretty intense pull that eases gradually after several steps. Maybe that's movement pain. An afternoon of errands leads to more pain that evening. Maybe that's overload pain. After a nearly sleepless night, he has a significant increase in his pain. Even his pant leg feels irritating. Maybe that's sensitivity pain.

His knee did not produce one mysterious problem four times. He experienced four patterns that called for four different considerations.

Keep reading because we are going to break each one down more so you can think about what kind of pain you might be experiencing.

How to Use This Information

Okay, how do you use this book? When pain shows up, and it is not fitting the description of something more serious that we just discussed, try asking these four questions about your pain:

1. Did it come with swelling and the general soreness of surgery?

2. Did it happen during one movement?
3. Did it show up later after more activity?
4. Did it feel unusually intense after poor sleep, stress, or repeated checking in with your knee?

Your answers may point strongly toward one pattern or show that two patterns overlap. That is already more useful than saying, "My pain is a seven," because now you are describing what happened around the pain.

Read the four pattern sections first. Then use the matching-strategies section to connect the likely pattern with options that commonly help. If the pain is new, severe, worsening, or paired with a warning sign, use the medical guidance in the warning-sign section above.

Surgical Pain

Surgical pain comes from the surgery itself, including the trauma to the knee and surrounding tissues along with the soreness and swelling that accompany healing. It is usually strongest early after surgery and gradually becomes less prominent over time, although the pace can look very different from one person to another.

The first several days after surgery are often the most uncomfortable. Pain medication, nerve blocks, and other pain-management strategies may all be part of the early plan your surgical team has given you. As a nerve block wears off or your activity increases, you may notice periods when the pain becomes more noticeable.

Over the first couple of weeks, many people notice some improvement, but soreness, swelling, and pain with activity can still be significant. Your knee is also being asked to do more during this time, so an easier morning and a more uncomfortable evening can both fit within the early surgical-pain pattern.

During the following weeks, surgical pain often continues to settle while movement and activity gradually increase. You may still have flare-ups, especially after a more demanding day, and your medication needs may change along the way. Follow the medication plan and any instructions your surgeon or other medical provider recommends.

By six weeks and beyond, many people have much less of the broad soreness associated with surgery, but pain can still vary widely. Some people improve quickly, while others follow a slower path. Your own trend over several weeks gives you much more useful information than trying to match one exact date on the calendar.

Friends or family may think you should be finished with pain by a certain week. Their expectations are not a measure of what you should feel. That may be difficult to manage. Remember, your pain is your experience, not theirs. Understanding your own pain gives you a stronger reference point than someone else's expectations.

This surgical pain pattern often feels broad rather than tied to one movement. Your knee may ache while you sit, feel heavy when you stand, or tighten as swelling increases throughout the day. Your incision may be sensitive, and the front of your knee may feel as if a strap is wrapped around it.

Swelling helps explain several of these sensations. More fluid around your knee leaves less room in and around the knee joint for easy bending. That is why your pants can feel comfortable in the morning and annoyingly tight around your knee by dinner, or later in the day after you've been standing up more.

Knee stiffness after sitting fits here too, especially when swelling is greater. You stand up after a meal, the first few steps feel wooden, and then your knee stiffness begins to ease. That familiar start-up pattern often coincides with surgical pain and swelling.

John notices the pattern early after surgery. He completes his exercises, stands while making dinner, and takes a few short walks around the house. By evening, his knee is fuller, tighter, and harder to bend. Nothing dramatic happened. He is still healing after surgery. Swelling simply built as the day went on.

His function can still be improving while these symptoms fluctuate. He may walk farther and stand longer even though swelling and soreness vary from day to day. Progress and pain do not always move in matching straight lines.

Think about the characteristics of this pain pattern. How long has it been since your surgery? Does this seem to match the type of pain you are experiencing now?

As swelling and surgical soreness become less prominent, some people find that movement, overload, or sensitivity explains more of what they feel. That change is one reason pain can seem to follow different rules over time.

Movement Pain

Movement pain is pain you can often connect to a specific action. Bending, straightening, standing up, walking, stairs, getting in the car, or rolling in bed are common examples, but not an exhaustive list. Fortunately, we move in many more ways than that. Your clue is the timing: the pain appears when you move.

Why can movement hurt? You are asking your knee joint to bend, straighten, support weight, and help control your body while strength, swelling, motion, and coordination are still changing. A tight pull at the end of a bend is more likely movement pain and different from a pain that starts after hours on your feet, which is more likely overload pain.

Movement is necessary after knee replacement. It helps you regain function and decrease the risk of blood clots and other post-surgical complications. Make sure you are participating in the movements your health care team has advised.

John used to treat every painful movement like a stop sign. If standing hurt once, he expected the next attempt to hurt too. Then he noticed that the first step often hurt most and the next several became easier.

That change during the movement is useful. Pain that eases after a few steps often behaves differently from pain that grows with every repetition and leaves your knee more swollen afterward.

What if you identify the movement, see whether the pain changes as you continue, and check how your knee responds afterward? If it settles near your usual level and your function is steady, the pattern may be movement pain rather than overload, which we will discuss next.

Movement pain can overlap with another pattern. Often it does. A swollen knee may hurt more when it bends. A long day may make stairs harder that evening. Poor sleep may make the same first step feel much sharper. Start with the movement, then look at what else changed to help you identify why you are having that particular pain and what you might do about it.

If you can say, "It hurts when I first stand, eases after several steps, and does not leave me more swollen later," you have already identified a useful pattern that may very well be movement pain. That description is far more useful than "standing hurts."

Think about the characteristics of the movement pain pattern. Does this seem to match the type of pain you are experiencing now?

Overload Pain

Overload pain starts after a long period of activity or waits until later to appear. You get through your exercises, errands, lunch out, or a family visit and think you did fine. Then your knee becomes more swollen and stiffer or feels harder to move that evening or the next morning, or both.

John runs into overload pain on his best-feeling days. For him, less pain feels like permission to make up for lost time. He walks farther, adds another errand, and finally handles the small job he has been postponing.

None of those activities feels excessive while he does them. But by dinner, his knee is swollen and difficult to bend. He starts looking for one guilty activity, but the walk, stairs, errands, and time on his feet all contributed to the total.

That total is the key.

All that activity adds up, even when it doesn't feel like much at the time. Exercise counts. Walking counts. Laundry, cooking, standing, stairs, and the extra trip across the store count too.

This often comes up during a physical therapy visit. Someone tells me they don't understand why they are sore and swollen in the morning. When I ask them to tell me about it, they say it didn't make sense. They hadn't done anything that should have caused it. They felt so great one morning that they vacuumed the entire house, went shopping, and then went out to dinner and for an evening walk. When they get done explaining it to me, that's when they realize they overdid it.

This is how the common boom-and-bust pattern develops. A good day leads to a large increase in activity. The delayed pain and swelling lead to a sharp decrease the next day. After several rounds, activity feels unpredictable even though the pattern itself is fairly consistent.

A familiar delayed pain response that gradually improves over time and eases toward your recent level often points to overload. A new change that keeps worsening is a different situation and belongs with the warning-sign guidance.

Try asking, "What did the whole day include?" A longer walk may have been fine on its own. The longer walk plus exercises, groceries, stairs, and dinner preparation may have crossed your current limit.

If the pain appeared later after a busier day, overload pain may be part of the answer. You now have something specific to adjust and observe.

Think about the characteristics of this pain pattern. Does this seem to match the type of pain you are experiencing now?

Sensitivity Pain

Sensitivity pain is often the hardest pattern to trust because the pain can feel out of proportion to what you did. You rested. You skipped the long walk. You did not spend the afternoon shopping. Yet your knee hurts more, feels more irritated, or refuses to fade into the background.

John notices it after a poor night of sleep. The skin around his knee feels unpleasant when his pant leg brushes it. At bedtime, the light pressure of the sheet feels irritating enough that he keeps moving the covers. The discomfort also reaches a wider area around the front and sides of his knee than usual.

Your brain creates the experience of pain by processing signals from your knee along with other information. Sleep, fatigue, stress, previous pain, expectations, and how often you check the area can change how strongly you experience those signals. This is a real, physical, nervous-system response.

I want to make sure the label for this category is clear. Sensitivity pain does not describe the individual as being sensitive. It describes a characteristic the nervous system is demonstrating. The role of a nerve is to send a signal. If we didn't have good sensitivity in the nerves that go to our fingers, we wouldn't be able to feel texture, manipulate small objects, or write. Nerves that function well are important.

Some sensations become harder to filter after surgery. A light touch that you would normally ignore may feel irritating. If you check your knee every few minutes because you are worried, your brain keeps receiving the message that the area may need protection. The symptom can become harder to tune out.

John compares several of these days. The worst ones often follow poor sleep, exhaustion, or hours spent worrying and repeatedly testing his knee. None is the only cause. Together, they add up and can explain why the same ordinary walk can feel tolerable one day and miserable the next.

Pain can also change how you approach a movement. After a painful movement happens several times, you may start bracing before you even try it again. You hold your breath, tighten your body, move cautiously, and watch for the pain. That preparation may make the movement feel harder and keep your focus locked on the symptom.

You may recognize sensitivity after poor sleep or a stressful day. Swelling or movement pain may still be present. Sensitivity helps explain why the volume seems turned up even though the physical activity did not increase much.

If the symptom returns toward your familiar level as sleep, fatigue, and repeated checking improve, that pattern gives you another clue about what may be contributing. The warning-sign section still applies to anything new, severe, or worsening.

Recognizing sensitivity lets you respond to the whole experience instead of assuming you must have damaged your knee. You can address sleep, tension, repeated checking, and irritating touch while still respecting the physical symptoms you're experiencing.

Think about the characteristics of this pain pattern. Does this seem to match the type of pain you are experiencing now?

Which Pain Pattern Fits What You're Feeling?

When pain increases, your first thought is usually, "What should I do?" Start one step earlier: "Which pattern does this look most like?" Think about the four patterns we just talked about and decide which pain pattern fits what you're feeling.

First, is your knee more swollen, warm, heavy, sore, or harder to bend as part of the general response to surgery? That points toward surgical pain.

Second, does the pain begin with one movement and change as you repeat it or continue walking? That points toward movement pain.

Third, did the pain or swelling appear later after a day with more exercise, walking, errands, stairs, or standing? That points toward overload pain.

Fourth, does the pain feel unusually strong or irritating after poor sleep, fatigue, stress, repeated checking, or contact from clothing or bedding? That points toward sensitivity pain.

Your answer may be "a little of two or three." That's fine. Start with the pattern that best explains the timing, then read the matching options in the next sections. If none fits, or the change is severe or worsening, move to the warning-sign guidance.

Keep in mind that the same activity can feel different as the weeks and months pass. Strength, movement, swelling, sleep, fatigue, and sensitivity all affect how your knee responds. You will see those differences throughout the next four sections.

John uses the questions after standing from his chair. The pain appears with the first step and eases after several more. There is no later increase in swelling. That sounds more like movement pain than overload, so he stops asking why and relaxes about the symptom and stops treating the whole day as ruined.

After errands, the pattern is different. His knee feels fine while he is out, then becomes swollen and harder to bend that evening. He recognizes overload and looks at the total day rather than blaming the last stair he climbed.

A pattern you recognize gives you a reasonable place to start and puts you in the driver's seat. You are using your own knowledge to make sense of your own pain, not just replacing one vague sentence with another. The goal may be to say, "This may be movement pain because it starts with the first step and eases," or, "This may be overload because it appeared three hours after a much busier day."

Matching Strategies to the Pain Pattern

Great work. You identified the pain pattern that seems to fit what you are experiencing. Now you can use that information to consider workable strategies that are commonly used for that pattern.

These are options to consider, not individual treatment instructions. Your medical history and your health care team's instructions still set the boundaries. You get to decide which options fit your situation, try a sensible strategy, and pay attention to how your knee responds.

For Surgical Pain: Swelling, Positioning, and Cold

When surgical pain is leading, cold therapy is usually the first place to start. It is one of the most useful strategies for early pain and swelling after knee replacement, and the 2026 APTA guideline supports its use. You might use an ice pack, cold wrap, or another cold therapy method that fits the instructions you were given. No single device, temperature, or schedule works for everyone, so use the method that fits your skin sensitivity, circulation, medical history, and current stage after surgery.

Next, pay attention to positioning. If your knee feels heavy, tight, swollen, or harder to bend, elevating your leg may help reduce some swelling. Early after surgery, guidelines also support elevated positioning as part of swelling management. Find a comfortable position and follow the instructions you were given. I've noticed that many people elevate their leg but don't get their knee above their heart. This can really make a difference. Sometimes a small change in how you rest makes your knee feel noticeably better.

Keep your knee moving too. Walking, bending, straightening, and the exercises already in your plan may make it easier to keep working toward better movement and function. On a more swollen or sore day, you may need to shorten a session, reduce repetitions, or give yourself more time between activities. Then pay attention to how you feel afterward.

Also consider your day as a whole. Early after surgery, it is easy to underestimate how much activity adds up. Walking to the bathroom, getting meals, doing exercises, taking a shower, going to appointments, and making extra trips around the house all count. If your knee is getting progressively more swollen, sore, or difficult to move as the day goes on, you might be doing more than it is ready to handle right now. Spread out your activity, take more breaks, and follow any walking or step limits your surgeon or rehabilitation team has given you.

Medication may also be part of the picture, especially earlier after surgery. Follow your surgeon's or other medical provider's medication plan, and use it alongside other strategies rather than expecting one tool to do everything.

Then step back and consider the whole response. Is the swelling settling? Is your knee moving more comfortably? Are you getting closer to your recent level after a harder part of the day? Compare your knee with your own recent days and weeks, not someone else's timeline.

Great work. You are paying attention to the pattern, choosing a strategy, and using the response to decide what comes next.

For Movement Pain: Change the Movement, Then Recheck

For movement pain, start by changing the movement itself. You can adjust the range, speed, position, or support and see whether that changes what you feel. A smaller bend, a slower pace, using your hands for support, or changing your position may make the movement easier without avoiding it altogether. Stay within any movement, weight-bearing, or exercise precautions your surgeon or rehabilitation team has given you.

Next, notice how much you are doing. Fewer repetitions, a shorter walking bout, or a little more time between efforts may be enough to keep the movement manageable. You can always build back up as your knee tolerates more.

A brief warm-up is useful too, especially when the first few movements feel the worst. A few gentle bends, short steps, or easier repetitions may help you get your knee moving before you ask more of yourself. If the movement becomes easier as you continue, that makes it easier for you to understand how your pain is behaving.

Then step back and look at the response without turning it into a test you repeat over and over. Notice whether the pain settles, whether the movement becomes easier, and whether your knee stays near its usual level afterward or becomes more swollen and sore later. Look for the overall response, not every sensation. Checking once or twice can give you useful information. Repeatedly bending, pressing, comparing, or testing your knee can keep your attention locked on the symptom and may contribute to sensitivity.

Use that response to guide the next choice. If a smaller range, slower pace, better support, or fewer repetitions makes the movement more manageable and your knee settles afterward, that may be a useful adjustment for now. If the pain keeps building, the movement becomes harder with each repetition, or your knee is noticeably more swollen or sore later, that is information too. You may need to change the amount, adjust how you do the movement, or give yourself more time before trying again.

One painful repetition doesn't have to decide everything. Review the pattern across the movement, the rest of the activity, and what happens afterward.

Great work. You are learning which adjustments help you move more comfortably, and which ones need to change. That gives you something much more useful than simply deciding that a movement "hurts" or "doesn't hurt."

For Overload Pain: Adjust the Total Day

For overload pain, start by looking back at the whole day. Think about everything your knee had to handle, not just the activity you were doing when you finally noticed the pain. Walking, exercises, errands, stairs, cooking, standing, household tasks, appointments, and social activities all count. One activity may have been completely reasonable on its own. The combination may simply have been more than your knee was ready to handle that day.

Once you see the total, pick one thing to change. Start with the easiest adjustment. You might shorten one outing, do fewer errands at once, move your exercises to a quieter part of the day, or take a break between two demanding activities. You do not need to redesign your entire schedule every time your knee gets irritated. One small shift may be enough to make the day more manageable.

Next, pay attention to how your activities are stacked together. Several moderate activities done back-to-back can sometimes create more trouble than one harder activity followed by a break. If you walk, exercise, shower, go shopping, and then stand to make a meal without much rest in between, you don't have much time to recover between activities. Spreading those activities out gives you a better chance to keep doing what you want without repeatedly ending the day with a large increase in swelling or soreness.

Pacing is especially useful here. Think of pacing as planning, not surrender. A good day may tempt you to catch up on everything at once, especially when you finally feel more like yourself. You can still take advantage of the good day. Just resist the urge to turn one better morning into a marathon of everything you have been putting off. Build the day in a way that lets you stay active without repeatedly overloading yourself.

Then give yourself some time before deciding whether the adjustment worked. Overload pain often shows up later, so the response may not be obvious right away. You might feel fine while you are active and notice more swelling, knee stiffness, soreness, or difficulty moving several hours later or the next morning. Look at that delayed response as information about the total amount your knee handled.

If the next evening or morning is closer to your usual level after you shorten, spread out, or rearrange activity, that is useful information. You may have found a better amount or arrangement for where your knee is right now. If the same large, delayed response keeps happening, make another small adjustment rather than blaming one random movement or giving up on the whole activity.

As your strength, motion, and endurance improve, you can gradually add more back in. Maybe the shorter shopping trip becomes longer. Two errands may become three. You might exercise and go out later in the same day without paying for it that evening. The goal is to learn what your knee can handle now and keep expanding gradually from there.

Great work. Overload pain gives you something concrete to work with. Step back and consider the whole day, choose one change, give your knee time to respond, and use that response to guide the next step. You are not trying to create a perfect day. You are learning how to arrange activity so you can do more of what matters to you with fewer big setbacks afterward.

For Sensitivity Pain: Reduce the Extra Irritation

For sensitivity pain, start with anything that may be adding extra irritation to the pain experience right now. Swelling, soreness, or movement pain may still be present at the same time. Sensitivity simply adds another part of the picture to consider.

First, notice obvious irritants. Is a pant leg rubbing the incision area? Are the sheets or blankets bothering your knee at night? Is one position putting pressure on an area that already feels irritated? Start with the easiest adjustments. Move the blanket, try a different position, adjust the clothing, or use softer material around the area. Small comfort adjustments may reduce irritation when your nervous system is already paying close attention to sensations from your knee.

Next, reduce how often you test your knee. It is very tempting to bend it again, press on the sore area, compare it with the other knee, or keep checking to see whether the pain is still there. A few checks may be enough to tell you what is happening. Repeating the same test over and over keeps bringing your attention back to the symptom. Give yourself some space between checks instead of searching for another update every few minutes.

Notice where your attention is going too. Pain naturally pulls your focus toward your knee, especially when the sensation is new or irritating. You might find yourself monitoring every step, every bend, or every shift in position. Direct your attention somewhere else for a while. Listen to music or a podcast, talk with someone, read, watch something you enjoy, or focus on another activity. You are not ignoring what you are feeling. You are giving your nervous system a break from constant surveillance.

Then, notice muscle tension. Pain often makes us brace without realizing it. You might tighten your thigh, grip the chair, hold your breath, clench your jaw, or stiffen your whole body before a movement you expect to hurt. Take a moment to loosen your grip, relax your shoulders and jaw, and slow your breathing. A few slow breaths may reduce some of that extra tension before you move.

Breathing is a surprisingly effective way to reduce some of the tension that builds around pain. When you expect a movement to hurt, you may hold your breath, tighten your muscles, and brace before you even begin. Slowing your breath gives you something simple to use before or during a difficult movement.

One option is the physiological sigh, sometimes called cyclic sighing when it is repeated. Take a deep breath in through your nose, then add a second, shorter inhale to fill your lungs a bit more. Breathe out slowly and completely through your mouth. One or two of these breaths may be enough before standing, walking, or another movement that has been making you tense. Research on cyclic sighing has also shown improvements in mood and a reduction in stress-related body responses.

Another option is diaphragmatic breathing. Let your abdomen expand as you breathe in, rather than lifting your shoulders and upper chest. Then exhale slowly and comfortably. The goal is not to force a huge breath. It is simply to breathe more slowly and with less tension.

Box breathing follows a simple rhythm: inhale, pause, exhale, pause, using roughly equal amounts of time for each part. For example, breathe in for four seconds, pause for four seconds, breathe out for four seconds, and pause again for four seconds. Some people like the structure because counting gives their attention somewhere else to go. If holding your breath feels uncomfortable, skip the pauses and instead use a slow inhale followed by an easy, longer exhale.

These techniques are not treatments for the knee itself. They are ways to reduce bracing, muscle tension, and stress-related body responses that may be adding to the pain experience. Use the method that feels comfortable and natural for you. If any breathing technique makes you feel lightheaded or uncomfortable, return to your normal breathing.

Consider how you approach a movement. If you expect the movement to hurt, guarding may begin before you even move. Set yourself up comfortably, breathe normally, and move at a controlled pace rather than rushing. This gives your body an opportunity to experience the movement without adding extra tension before it starts.

After you reduce some of that guarding, practice with a movement that already feels familiar and manageable. Choose something you already know, and that feels comfortable enough, rather than repeatedly testing the motion that worries you most. A short walk, gentle bending and straightening, or another familiar exercise from your plan may allow movement to feel more ordinary instead of turning every repetition into an examination. Keep it simple and give yourself time to settle into it.

Sensitivity can also show up with touch. If clothing, bedding, or light contact feels unusually irritating, make the environment more comfortable rather than repeatedly rubbing or testing the area. As the irritation settles, normal contact may gradually become easier to tolerate. The goal is for everyday touch to demand less of your attention.

Now consider the whole day. Poor sleep, exhaustion, stress, and spending a lot of time focused on your knee may increase pain intensity. A bad night of sleep or a stressful day isn't always something you control, but recognizing its role gives you another piece of the picture. After very poor sleep, a quieter day, familiar movement, and fewer repeated checks may fit better than assuming something suddenly went wrong.

If sleep has been difficult, focus on the parts you can influence. Make the room and bedding comfortable, settle into a position that works for you, and use the pain-management plan already available to you. Give yourself time to wind down rather than spending the last part of the evening repeatedly checking your knee or searching for signs that something is different.

Pain often seems louder at night because less is competing for your attention. During the day, you may be talking with someone, watching television, moving around, or thinking about other things. At 2:00 a.m., your knee may feel like the only thing in the room. Swelling from the day, staying in one position longer, medication timing, and disrupted sleep may all contribute to that experience.

The whole night pattern may point to what deserves attention first, whether that is swelling, position, sleep setup, a medication-timing question to discuss with your healthcare provider, or simply how much attention you are giving your knee.

The same idea applies during a stressful day. You may not be able to remove the stress, but you can control how much time you spend focused on your knee. Give yourself periods when it is not the main topic. Listen to something, read, talk with someone, work on a hobby, or let your attention go somewhere else for a while.

If several of these factors are present at once, pick one or two to address first. The easiest place to start might be making the bedding more comfortable and checking your knee less often. Another option is to take a few slow breaths before standing and use a familiar movement instead of repeatedly testing the painful one. You don't need to work on everything at once. Start with what seems most relevant and easiest to address.

Give those adjustments some time before deciding whether they worked. Notice the overall pattern rather than checking every few minutes. Does the clothing or bedding become easier to tolerate? Does the movement feel less threatening? Are you bracing less? Does the pain begin to settle as fatigue, tension, or repeated checking decrease? Those responses may give you a better sense of how much sensitivity is contributing.

Sensitivity often overlaps with the other pain patterns, so continue addressing swelling, movement, and activity load when those are present too. Cold therapy may fit when swelling is prominent. A painful movement may need an adjustment. A demanding day may need less activity or more spacing between tasks. At the same time, you may address sensitivity by reducing repeated checking, tension, and unnecessary irritation. These strategies work together and give you several ways to respond to what you are experiencing.

Great work. Sensitivity pain often feels especially frustrating because the intensity may vary even when your activity has stayed about the same. Now you have several options:

reduce unnecessary irritation, check your knee less often, shift your attention away from constant monitoring, release tension around movement, use familiar movement, and consider the effects of sleep, fatigue, and stress.

You get to choose where to start, make one or two workable adjustments, and give your nervous system time to respond.

When More Than One Pain Pattern Fits

Some days your knee may seem to be doing several things at once, and that can be incredibly frustrating. You may think you finally understand what is causing the pain, only to notice something different later in the day. More than one pain pattern can be happening at the same time. Your knee may be swollen, hurt with bending, become more irritated after a busy day, and feel even more uncomfortable after a poor night of sleep.

And honestly, that is what real life often looks like. Pain does not always arrive neatly labeled as one thing at a time. Your day includes movement, activity, sleep, stress, swelling, fatigue, and a hundred other variables mixed together. The goal is to make enough sense of the pattern that you have a place to start, not to force every symptom into one perfect category.

Start by putting the events in order. What happened first? Swelling may have already been present in the morning. Stairs brought on movement pain later. A busy afternoon added overload, and poor sleep increased sensitivity overnight. Seeing the sequence can make a complicated pain day much easier to understand.

Try this with your own day. Think back over the last several hours. What was already present when you woke up? What happened when you moved? What showed up later? What felt more irritating after fatigue or poor sleep? You are not trying to perform a perfect analysis. You are simply putting the pieces in order.

Here is one example. Your knee is already swollen and stiff in the morning, so bending feels uncomfortable. You go to an appointment, walk more than usual, and then notice even more swelling that evening. In that situation, surgical pain and overload may both be contributing. You may use the swelling-management strategies that fit your instructions and also make the next day less demanding.

Or the main problem may start with one movement. Standing from a chair hurts sharply at first, but the pain eases after a few steps. Later that day, after errands and exercises, your knee becomes more swollen and sore. The first part may fit movement pain, while the later response may fit overload. You can adjust the movement and also consider the total amount you did that day.

Sensitivity can layer on top of either pattern. Your knee may be mildly swollen and sore, but after a poor night of sleep the same pain feels much stronger. Your pant leg bothers you; you notice yourself checking your knee more often, and every movement suddenly seems more irritating. The swelling may still be real, but sensitivity may be turning up the intensity. In that situation, you can still address the swelling while also reducing repeated checking, muscle tension, and other extra irritants.

The leading pattern might also shift during the day. Surgical pain may be more noticeable in the morning. Movement pain may show up on the stairs. Overload may appear in the evening. Sensitivity may become more obvious overnight when you are tired and trying to sleep. You do not need to force the whole day into one category.

When several patterns fit, start with the part that seems most relevant and easiest to address right now. If swelling is prominent, use the swelling-management strategies that fit your instructions. If one movement is especially painful, adjust the movement. If the day became much busier than usual, reduce or rearrange the total activity. If sensitivity seems to add extra irritation, work on what may be turning up the volume on the pain experience.

You can address more than one part at a time, but you do not have to tackle everything at once. In fact, making one or two modest adjustments may give you better information than trying six things and then wondering what helped. Start with the pattern that seems to explain the biggest part of the problem and build from there.

Then give yourself some time and look at the overall response. Did the swelling settle? Did the movement become easier? Did the delayed soreness improve after you adjusted the total day? Did the pain become less irritating after better sleep or less repeated checking? Those responses can help you see which part of the pattern was most influential.

This is where the framework starts becoming useful in everyday life. You are not looking for a perfect label. You sort through the pieces, choose a place to start, and respond as the situation unfolds. That is a much more useful way to handle a complicated pain day than treating every increase in pain like one big mystery.

You now have information, structure, and a way to work through this. Trust yourself enough to use it. You know more about your pain than you did before, and that gives you somewhere to begin.

What Else Can Help?

The four pain patterns give you a strong starting point, and now you can build on that. Once you have an idea of what may be driving the pain, other strategies may support what you are already doing and give you more confidence about the next step.

Some options focus on gradually building tolerance for activity. Others provide short-term relief, make sleep easier, reduce irritation, or make movement and daily life more comfortable. You do not need every strategy. Think of this as a toolkit, with different options serving different purposes at different times.

The important part is understanding what each strategy is meant to do. Temporary relief still has value. A strategy that makes movement more comfortable may also be worthwhile. Consider the benefit, the evidence behind it, and how it fits your situation, then decide whether it belongs in your plan.

As you read through the next sections, think of these as additional options rather than requirements. Some may fit now. Others may fit later. A few may not fit you at all. That is okay. The purpose of this section is to give you more ways to respond to pain with greater confidence, flexibility, and understanding.

Why Building Tolerance Helps

As you get farther along after knee replacement, the way you manage pain starts to shift. Early on, much of your attention goes toward swelling, medication, positioning, and getting through the basics of the day. Later, gradually increasing what you are able to do becomes an important part of managing pain.

That is what building tolerance means. You work with an activity that is still uncomfortable at a level you currently manage, then gradually add more over time. As your tolerance improves, the activity often feels easier, less irritating, and less likely to take over the rest of your day.

Walking for ten minutes might still leave you aching. You stay with that amount for a while, and eventually ten minutes feels more routine. Then you add more. Stairs might still be difficult, but you notice that you use the railing less or move with more control. You might stand in the kitchen longer before pain pulls your attention away from what you are doing.

That is how progress starts to build.

Research supports gradually increasing activity after knee replacement while considering pain, swelling, function, safety, and your overall response. In everyday language, you challenge yourself enough to build strength and endurance without repeatedly pushing beyond what you tolerate well. Your response afterward guides the next step.

The same activity will not feel identical every day. John notices this during one of his regular walks. After a good night of sleep and a quieter morning, the walk feels routine. On another day, he has already run errands, slept poorly, and spent more time on his feet. The same route feels much harder.

The route is the same. The day around it is different.

One painful day doesn't tell the whole story. Think about what has happened over several weeks. Are you walking farther before pain appears? Does it settle more quickly afterward? Are you standing longer, moving more easily, or getting through more of the day before pain becomes hard to ignore?

Those are signs of progress, even when pain has not disappeared.

Different activities also progress at different rates. Walking might feel fairly comfortable while stairs remain difficult. You might shop longer but still feel stiff after sitting through dinner. A workout might go well while standing in one place for a long time remains uncomfortable. All of that fits with rebuilding your tolerance for everyday activity.

A good day can make it easy to do too much. Less pain often makes it tempting to catch up on everything you have been putting off. You walk farther, add another errand, do your exercises, and decide to tackle one more task while you are feeling good. A few hours later, pain or swelling increases.

That experience still teaches you something. It shows what felt manageable in the moment and where the total amount may have become too much for that day.

Smaller increases are usually easier to judge. Add some activity, then notice how you feel afterward. If the pain stays manageable and your symptoms return toward your recent level, continue building from there. If pain and swelling remain elevated, reduce the amount and try again another day.

It can be hard to be patient when you are ready to get back to the things you actually want to do. That may mean walking, climbing stairs, shopping, gardening, traveling, exercising, playing with your grandkids, or standing long enough to cook dinner without thinking about your knee every five minutes. You are gradually building your ability to do more of those things.

Progress is not measured only by whether pain is still present. Ask yourself what you are doing now that was harder a few weeks ago. Pain might show up later, feel less intense, settle faster, or interfere with fewer activities. You might simply get through more of the day before it becomes noticeable.

That is progress.

Building tolerance allows pain to take up less space in your life. Over time, you become stronger, more capable, and more comfortable with everyday activity. Things that once felt difficult or intimidating begin to feel ordinary again.

That is where you are headed.

Hands-On Care: Short-Term Relief and Movement

Hands-on care may help some people feel more comfortable, especially when stiffness, muscle guarding, or soreness is making movement harder. Massage, soft-tissue work, or joint-based techniques may temporarily reduce pain or make movement feel easier.

That relief can be useful. If hands-on care helps you move more comfortably, sleep better, or participate more easily in exercise and daily activity, it may be a great part of the bigger plan.

The important thing is to keep the role of hands-on care in perspective. It may settle symptoms for a while, but the longer-term changes usually come from gradually rebuilding movement, strength, and tolerance. Think of hands-on care as something that may open the door so you can keep doing the work that helps you move forward.

TENS: Another Option for Temporary Pain Relief

TENS, or transcutaneous electrical nerve stimulation, is another option some people use for short-term pain relief. The small electrical impulses can change how pain feels for some people while the unit is being used.

TENS is not appropriate for everyone, and important precautions apply to medical conditions, implanted devices, skin sensation, electrode placement, and where the unit is used. Talk with your surgeon, physical therapist, or another qualified healthcare professional before trying TENS so they can tell you whether it is appropriate for you and how to use it safely.

If TENS helps you feel more comfortable, it may make it easier to rest, move, or get through an exercise session. Benefits vary from person to person, and research after knee replacement is still limited.

Think of TENS as another tool you may decide to try rather than something your progress depends on. If it gives you useful relief, great. If it does very little for you, you haven't missed an essential part of your rehab.

Taping: A Supportive Tool for Some People

Taping may help some people feel more supported or comfortable during movement. Different taping techniques serve different purposes, and how the tape is applied may change how your skin, muscles, or knee feel during walking or exercise.

A physical therapist can help you decide whether taping is worth trying and which technique best fits your situation. They can also show you where to place the tape, how much tension to use, and what to watch for if your skin becomes irritated.

For some people, that extra support or change in sensation is worthwhile. For others, it makes little difference. Evidence is limited, so think of taping as a supportive option rather than a primary treatment for pain.

If taping helps you move more comfortably or feel more confident with an activity, that can still be worthwhile. Use it as one tool alongside the bigger pieces of your rehabilitation, including movement, strength, activity progression, and the strategies that fit your pain pattern.

Medication and Non-Prescription Products: Part of the Pain Plan

Medication can be an important part of pain management after knee replacement, especially in the earlier weeks. Your surgeon or other medical provider may recommend prescription medication, over-the-counter medication, or both. Follow the plan they gave you. This book cannot tell you which medication to take, how much to take, when to take it, or when to stop it.

Also remember that products sold without a prescription may still act like medications in your body. Acetaminophen, anti-inflammatory medications, sleep aids, topical pain products, and many supplements interact with other medications or affect medical conditions. "Over the counter" does not mean "risk-free."

If you are thinking about adding something new, changing the timing, taking less, taking more, or stopping something, talk with the healthcare professional who knows your medical history and current medications. Your surgeon, primary care provider, or pharmacist can assist you in sorting out what is appropriate for you.

Bring the exact product name with you when you ask. "A pain reliever," "a sleep aid," or "a supplement" is not enough information. The active ingredients and dose matter, and some combination products contain more than one medication.

Topical products deserve the same caution. Creams, gels, patches, and other products may provide temporary relief, but skin around a recent incision may still be sensitive. Follow the instructions you were given about what you can safely apply to or near the surgical area.

Supplements may seem simple to add, but they still deserve caution. Products marketed for inflammation, joint pain, sleep, or healing may sound harmless because they are sold without a prescription, but they still contain active ingredients and may interact with prescription medications or health conditions. Make sure your medical team knows what you are taking.

For some people, medication makes it easier to sleep, move, exercise, or get through a difficult part of the day. That relief can be very useful. It is still one part of the larger pain picture. Feeling better after taking medication tells you that the medication decreased your pain. It does not tell you exactly which pain pattern was responsible or how much activity your knee is ready to handle next.

Use medication and non-prescription products as part of the larger plan your healthcare team has helped you build. Keep working with movement, swelling management, activity progression, sleep, and the strategies that fit your pain pattern.

When you have a medication question, ask. A pharmacist can be an excellent resource for questions about ingredients, interactions, and over-the-counter products, while your surgeon or other medical provider should guide changes to the prescription plan they have given you.

When a Strategy Helps One Day and Not the Next

One of the frustrating things about pain after knee replacement is that something can work really well one day and seem almost useless the next. You finally find something that gives you relief, and naturally you want to know why it worked and whether to count on it again.

Pain relief can be pretty convincing. Cold numbs your pain, and you think, "Okay, it must have been the swelling." Massage feels good, and suddenly that tight muscle seems like the whole explanation. Medication takes effect, and you breathe a sigh of relief. Those responses are useful, but pain usually has more than one contributor.

If something helps, take the win. Feeling better for a while might make it easier to move, sleep, exercise, or simply enjoy your day. It also gives you information about what may be contributing to the pain. One strategy that helps doesn't explain the whole pain experience.

You may also notice that a strategy that worked beautifully yesterday barely seems to make a difference today. Your cold pack did the trick Monday night and does nothing on Wednesday. A walk loosened your knee up yesterday, but today the same walk feels harder. Changing position helped you sleep one night and did very little the next.

Look at what else may be different today. Your knee may be more swollen, you may have slept poorly, spent more time on your feet, had a busier day, or simply be more tired or stressed. Those differences can affect how pain feels from one day to the next. The strategy may be the same, but your body is responding differently.

The reverse might happen too. Something that once bothered you may gradually become easier. A movement that used to make you brace may start to feel routine. A walk that once left your knee sore may eventually become part of an ordinary day. Your strength, movement, confidence, and tolerance are changing, so your response can change too.

Give yourself permission to use what works without needing it to prove exactly why you hurt. Relief is valuable all by itself. Then keep looking at the bigger pattern: what you did, how your knee responded, and what you felt over the next several hours or days.

A strategy can be useful without explaining everything. Sometimes it gives you a little relief, sometimes a lot, and sometimes almost none. What matters is that you now have another piece of information about how your knee responds. Over time, you may start to notice which strategies tend to work, when they help most, and when a different strategy may fit better.

When You Need More Help Sorting Out the Pain

Sometimes you can make sense of the pattern on your own. Other times, the pain behaves differently, several things seem to be happening at once, or you simply want another perspective. That is a good time to talk with your healthcare provider and give them a clear picture of what you have been experiencing.

A pain number tells only one part of the story. Saying, "My pain is a seven," tells your provider how intense it feels. Adding when it started, what you were doing, what happened next, and whether anything else showed up gives them much more context.

You might say, "The pain is strongest when I first stand up, then it eases after several steps." Or, "I felt pretty good while I was out running errands, but a few hours later my knee became more swollen and harder to bend." Those descriptions show your provider how the pain behaves instead of giving them only a number.

Let them know when the pain starts and what happens around it. Does it begin with a movement? Build as the day goes on? Show up later after more activity? Feel stronger after poor sleep or a stressful day? Include what you were doing before the pain increased and what happened afterward.

Also mention other symptoms you noticed. Swelling, warmth, redness, drainage, calf pain or swelling, a sudden loss of function, or difficulty putting weight on your leg can all be important. If something feels distinctly different from your usual experience, say that too.

Tell them what you have already tried. Cold therapy may have reduced the swelling. Adjusting the movement may have made it easier. Shortening a busy day may have reduced the delayed soreness. That gives your provider more context without assuming that one strategy explains the whole problem.

You do not have to walk in with the diagnosis figured out. You are simply bringing a specific description of what you are experiencing. The more detail you can give about timing, activity, other symptoms, and what happened next, the easier it is for your healthcare provider to understand the situation and guide the next step.

Reach out to your healthcare team. That is what they are there for. If something feels different, confusing, or concerning, bring it up. Asking questions about your pain doesn't bother anyone, and a specific description gives them a better starting point.

Decreased Pain Is Not the Only Sign of Progress

Pain is one way to measure how your knee is doing, but it is only one part of the picture. You may still have pain and be making meaningful progress at the same time.

Maybe you are walking farther before the pain starts. Maybe you stand longer, go up the stairs with more control, get through the grocery store with fewer breaks, or sleep for a longer stretch before pain wakes you up. Maybe you still have soreness after a busy day, but it settles faster than it did a few weeks ago.

Those changes count.

It can be easy to miss them when pain is still getting your attention. A difficult day may make it feel like nothing is getting better, even though your function has been improving in the background.

Try looking back over several weeks instead of judging everything by today. What can you do now that was harder before? Are you using less assistance? Moving with more confidence? Thinking about your knee less often during ordinary activities? Getting back to more of the things you enjoy?

Progress may also show up in how quickly you recover after activity. Maybe a busy afternoon used to leave you sore and swollen until the next day, and now your knee settles by evening. Stairs might still hurt, but they no longer feel like a major event. Maybe you can do more before the pain asks for your attention.

Pain may still be part of the process as your knee becomes stronger, more capable, and more reliable in everyday life. Keep an eye on the bigger picture. The changes you are looking for may be happening in your walking, endurance, confidence, sleep, independence, and ability to get back to your life.

That is progress too.

Common Traps That Make Pain Harder to Understand

Pain after knee replacement can be frustrating enough on its own. Then your brain starts trying to explain it, predict it, compare it, and occasionally turn one rough afternoon into a full documentary about everything that is going wrong.

That is a very human response.

The trouble starts when one painful moment gets more meaning than it deserves. A sore day becomes "I am going backward." One painful movement becomes "I damaged something." A friend who is doing better becomes proof that you are behind. Before long, the pain is still there, and now you are also carrying a whole pile of conclusions around with it.

The next few sections look at some of the most common traps people fall into while trying to make sense of pain. You may recognize one or two. You may recognize all of them. The point is not to catch yourself doing something wrong. It is to notice when a pattern is making the pain harder to understand and give yourself another way to respond.

A little perspective can go a long way here.

The Good-Day Trap

A good day can be incredibly convincing. Your knee feels better, the swelling is down, and suddenly everything you have been putting off starts looking manageable. So, you walk a little farther, add another errand, do some housework, finish your exercises, and then squeeze in one more thing because you are already up and moving.

By evening, you may notice more pain, swelling, or stiffness than you expected. This is one of the easiest ways overload sneaks in. The problem is usually not one activity. It is the way several activities stack together when you are feeling good. Less pain can make it seem like your knee has unlimited capacity for the day, even though it may still be building endurance.

A good day is still a good day. Enjoy it. Use it. Do more of what you want to do. Just give yourself enough time between activities to see how the day is adding up. That might mean choosing the longer walk and skipping the extra errand or doing the errands and saving the heavier household job for tomorrow. Spreading things out can help you enjoy the better day without setting yourself up for a large, delayed response later.

If you notice a familiar increase in swelling, soreness, or knee stiffness later that evening or the next morning, look back at the total day. Chances are, that familiar delayed response tells you how much activity you handled that day. It is not necessarily a formal complaint against one innocent trip to the grocery store.

As your tolerance improves, those better days will naturally hold more activity. For now, the goal is to enjoy the good days and build on them without turning every one into a catch-up day.

Judging Today Against Yesterday

Yesterday is a pretty unfair measuring stick for today. Maybe Tuesday felt surprisingly good, so when Wednesday hurts more, it can feel like something went wrong. But Wednesday may also include worse sleep, more standing, a harder therapy session, an appointment, or just a busier day overall.

That is why one-day comparisons can be misleading. Pain changes with activity, swelling, fatigue, sleep, stress, sitting, standing, and how much attention you are giving your knee. Two days that look similar on the calendar may feel very different to your knee.

Looking back over several weeks usually gives you a much clearer picture. Are you walking farther? Standing longer? Sleeping better? Getting through more of the day before pain starts demanding your attention? Is the pain settling faster after activity than it used to?

One rough day might feel discouraging, especially after a good one. It helps to remember that progress rarely moves in a perfectly straight line. A harder day can still fit within an overall trend moving in the right direction.

So, when today feels worse than yesterday, widen the lens slightly. You are allowed to have an off day without erasing the progress you have already made.

Treating Every Painful Movement as a Damage Test

A painful movement can feel like a verdict. You stand up, take a step, or bend your knee and immediately think, "I must have done something wrong." Once that thought takes hold, the next movement can start to feel like a test you have to pass.

One painful moment rarely tells the whole story. You already know that pain can change with swelling, stiffness, fatigue, sensitivity, and the demands of the day. The same movement may feel different a few minutes later, later that day, or on another day entirely.

The trap is treating every painful movement as proof that something has been damaged. That can make you brace, hesitate, or avoid a movement that may simply be uncomfortable right now. Pain gives you information, but it is only one piece of the picture.

If the pain feels distinctly different from your usual pattern, keeps worsening, or comes with a warning sign, that deserves more attention. Otherwise, one painful repetition can simply be one data point in a much bigger picture. You do not have to let one awkward step, or one difficult bend, decide what the whole day means.

Testing Your Knee Over and Over

Worry can turn you into a full-time knee inspector. You bend it again to see whether it still hurts, press on the sore spot, compare it with the other knee, or take a few more steps just to check. Before long, you have gathered a lot of information that may not actually be useful in making a decision.

Each test adds a little more movement and keeps your attention focused on your knee. Small changes become easier to notice, and normal ups and downs start to feel much bigger because you are checking so often. If the area is already sensitive, repeated testing can also add more irritation.

There are times when checking is useful. If you are trying to see whether a change in position helped, whether a movement is settling, or whether a symptom is getting worse, one or two checks may give you what you need. Repeating the same test every few minutes usually creates more noise than clarity.

Give yourself a little breathing room between checks. Let the activity, movement, or strategy have time to work before you test it again. You may find that the pattern becomes much easier to understand when you are not checking for an update every five minutes.

Changing Everything After One Difficult Day

One rough day can make you want to change everything. You cut back on walking, stop several exercises, avoid the movement that bothered you, change your routine, and start wondering whether you need to rebuild the whole plan. That reaction makes sense when your knee suddenly feels worse.

The problem is that changing six things at once makes the next day harder to interpret. If the pain improves, you won't know which change worked. If it stays the same, you still do not know whether your symptoms were simply settling after a difficult day.

A more useful approach is to make one or two reasonable changes that fit the pattern you are seeing. That may mean adjusting the total activity, changing one movement, using your swelling-management strategies, or giving sensitivity less fuel. Then give yourself enough time to see how you respond before you overhaul something else.

A difficult day can still teach you something without forcing you to start over. Look at what happened, make the adjustment that fits best, and let the next day give you more information. That keeps one bad day from turning into a complete rewrite of your whole rehab plan.

Searching for One Perfect Cause

Pain after knee replacement often has more than one contributing factor. Swelling may alter the way you move. A busy day may leave you with more swelling. Poor sleep may increase sensitivity, and worrying about a movement might make you tense before you even begin.

It is tempting to keep searching for one explanation that ties everything together. Sometimes there is an obvious reason. Other times, several smaller factors line up and create a much bigger pain day than any one of them would have caused alone.

Pain relief can give you useful information without giving you the whole answer. Cold may feel good even when swelling is only one piece of the problem. A different position may feel better even when movement isn't the only factor. One strategy may ease the pain without identifying a single cause.

You do not need a perfect explanation before trying an adjustment. A few clues about the timing and overall pattern may be enough to point you toward a place to start. Then pay attention to how you respond and build from there.

Comparing Your Timeline With Someone Else's

It is almost impossible not to compare. Someone tells you they were walking a mile at four weeks, driving at three weeks, or barely using pain medication by a certain date, and suddenly your own progress seems lackluster.

The problem is that you are comparing two completely different knees, bodies, histories, and lives. Strength before surgery, medical conditions, swelling, pain sensitivity, sleep, support at home, daily responsibilities, and how much activity someone does can all affect progress.

Two people can be at the same point on the calendar and still have very different pain, swelling, walking tolerance, sleep, and function. Progress can look very different from one person to another, even at the same stage after surgery.

Your own recent progress gives you much more useful information. Notice what has changed for you over the last few weeks. Maybe you are walking farther, moving more comfortably, sleeping longer, needing less help, or getting through more of the day before pain starts demanding your attention.

Other people can be encouraging, and their stories can give you ideas about what may be possible. Their experiences may be interesting, motivating, or reassuring, but your knee still follows its own course. Your progress is best judged by what changes for you over time.

Using Pain as the Only Scorecard

Pain has a way of grabbing the microphone. If it is louder today, it can make everything else that is going well feel less important. You may have walked farther, handled the stairs better, slept longer, or needed less help, but the pain is the thing that gets all the attention.

That makes a difficult day feel much worse than the bigger picture actually looks. Your knee can still be getting stronger and more capable while pain continues to come and go. Function, endurance, confidence, sleep, and how quickly your knee settles after activity may all be changing at the same time.

John catches himself doing this after a rough afternoon. His first thought is that he is getting nowhere because his knee hurts more. Then he realizes he just spent an hour shopping, carried groceries into the house, and stood long enough to make dinner, things that would have been much harder for him a few weeks earlier.

Pain still deserves your attention. It is useful information, and sometimes it tells you that something needs to change. It doesn't have to erase every other sign that your knee is moving forward.

When you think about the whole picture, you might find that pain is only one part of the story. And sometimes the rest of the story is going pretty well.

Quick Reference: What Am I Feeling?

Use this section when you want the short version. Maybe your pain changed, you are trying to sort out what pattern fits, or you simply want something you can glance at without rereading the whole chapter. Start with the closest pattern, use the matching strategy within the instructions you have been given, and move to the warning-sign guidance if the change is new, severe, steadily worsening, or distinctly different from what you usually experience.

Four Questions Before You Choose a Response

Is your knee generally swollen, warm, heavy, sore, or harder to bend, and was your surgery recent? Think **surgical pain**.

Does one movement bring on the pain, and does it change as you continue? Think **movement pain**.

Did the pain or swelling appear later after a busier day? Think **overload pain**.

Does the pain feel unusually strong after poor sleep, stress, repeated checking, or irritating touch? Think **sensitivity pain**.

Surgical Pain

Common clues include general soreness, pressure, heaviness, warmth, swelling, incision sensitivity, knee stiffness, or a band-like feeling around the front of the knee.

Common strategies include cold therapy, elevation, your medication plan, movement, and adjusting your day when activity increases swelling.

Movement Pain

The pain starts with a specific movement such as bending, straightening, standing, walking, or stairs.

Try changing one part of the movement, such as the range, speed, support, position, or number of repetitions. Then give yourself time to see how you respond.

Overload Pain

The activity may feel fine while you are doing it, but pain, swelling, knee stiffness, or difficulty moving shows up later that day or the next morning.

Look at the whole day. Shorten, spread out, or rearrange activity so you don't stack several demanding tasks together.

Sensitivity Pain

The pain may feel unusually strong or irritating. Clothing or bedding may bother the skin, or a familiar movement may feel much worse after poor sleep, fatigue, stress, or repeated checking.

Reduce unnecessary irritation, check your knee less often, release tension around movement, use a breathing technique such as a physiological sigh or slow diaphragmatic breathing, improve the sleep setup, and return to familiar movement that feels comfortable.

When More Than One Pattern Fits

More than one pattern can be happening at the same time. Put the events in order, start with the part that seems most relevant or changeable, and address more than one pattern when that makes sense.

When You Need More Help Sorting It Out

Give your healthcare provider a clear description of what happened: when the pain started, what you were doing, what changed, what other symptoms you noticed, and what happened afterward. Let them know whether the pattern feels familiar or distinctly different.

When to Skip the Pattern Questions

Seek medical attention for increasing redness or warmth, drainage, fever, worsening calf pain or swelling, sudden shortness of breath, chest discomfort, lightheadedness, a sudden major change after a fall or injury, or new difficulty putting weight on your leg.

A symptom that feels distinctly different from your usual pattern or continues to worsen also deserves medical evaluation.

Quick Reference: Pain Patterns

Simplified summary. For context, refer to the sections above.

Type	Feels Like	What People Try
Surgical	Swelling, tightness, pressure, constant awareness	Change positions, elevate, shorter time on feet, spread activity across the day, vary positions
Movement	Discomfort with bending, walking, standing	Keep moving if it settles, use smaller ranges, repeat with pauses, use short frequent movement
Overload	Feels okay during the day, worse later or next day	Break activity up, avoid big spikes, use step count, keep days more consistent
Sensitivity	Feels different, more intense, less predictable	Physiological sigh or slow breathing, attention shift, familiar movement, reducing irritation, sleep, and less repeated checking

Final Thoughts

Pain after knee replacement can be frustrating, exhausting, and unpredictable. Some days will make sense. Other days may leave you wondering why your knee suddenly feels different again.

You have more tools now to sort through those days. You can identify the pattern, choose a strategy that fits, notice the overall response, and ask for help when something feels different or concerning. You don't have to solve every painful moment perfectly to make good decisions about what comes next.

You may also start noticing that pain is no longer the only thing you pay attention to. Walking gets easier. Stairs feel more familiar. You stay on your feet longer, sleep better, and get through more of the day without thinking about your knee as much.

I want this book to help you make sense of your pain, so it feels less mysterious and overwhelming. I want you to understand what you are experiencing well enough to make thoughtful choices, know when to work with your team, and keep moving toward what matters most to you.

Ultimately, this is about getting back to living your life. Spending time with the people you love. Going places. Moving more freely. Returning to the activities that make you feel like yourself again. Keep moving toward that life, one good decision and one ordinary day at a time.

Continue Learning with Total Knee Success

Visit TotalKneeSuccess.com

There you'll find:

The **Total Knee Success Podcast™**, with practical education for every stage after knee replacement.

Walking Like Yourself Again After Knee Replacement, a book focused on walking, movement, and getting back to a more natural stride.

The **Total Knee Success™ Insider Newsletter**, with ongoing education, new resources, and updates for people at different stages after surgery.

If this book was helpful, an honest review on Amazon can inform other readers so they can decide whether it may be useful for them too. Thank you for being part of Total Knee Success™.

About the Author

Michelle Losurdo, PT, DPT, OCS, is a physical therapist and Board-Certified Clinical Specialist in Orthopaedic Physical Therapy with a special interest in total knee replacement rehabilitation.

She created and hosts the Total Knee Success Podcast™, where she helps people better understand pain, knee stiffness, swelling, walking, sleep, and the many questions that come up during rehabilitation after knee replacement.

Michelle is known for taking complicated rehabilitation and pain science concepts and explaining them in clear, conversational language. Her goal is for people to understand what they are experiencing, feel more confident asking questions, and make informed choices as they work toward getting back to the activities and routines they enjoy.

Visit TotalKneeSuccess.com for podcast episodes, educational resources, and additional education for life before and after knee replacement.

References

1. Bove AM, Carroll LA, Cone S, et al. Clinical practice guideline for physical therapist management of total knee arthroplasty: revision 2026. Phys Ther. 2026;106(7):pzag058. doi:10.1093/ptj/pzag058

2. Wylde V, Beswick A, Bruce J, Blom AW, Howells N, Gooberman-Hill R. Chronic pain after total knee arthroplasty. EFORT Open Rev. 2018;3(8):461-470. doi:10.1302/2058-5241.3.180004

3. Bertram W, Howells N, White SP, et al. Prevalence and patterns of neuropathic pain in people with chronic post-surgical pain after total knee arthroplasty. Bone Joint J. 2024;106-B(6):582-588. doi:10.1302/0301-620X.106B6.BJJ-2023-0889.R1

4. Kehlet H, Jensen TS, Woolf CJ. Persistent postsurgical pain: risk factors and prevention. Lancet. 2006;367(9522):1618-1625. doi:10.1016/S0140-6736(06)68700-X

5. Woolf CJ. Central sensitization: implications for the diagnosis and treatment of pain. Pain. 2011;152(3 suppl):S2-S15. doi:10.1016/j.pain.2010.09.030

6. Kim MS, Kim JJ, Kang KH, Kim MJ, In Y. Diagnosis of central sensitization and its effects on postoperative

outcomes following total knee arthroplasty: a systematic review and meta-analysis. Diagnostics (Basel). 2022;12(5):1248. doi:10.3390/diagnostics12051248

7. Finan PH, Goodin BR, Smith MT. The association of sleep and pain: an update and a path forward. J Pain. 2013;14(12):1539-1552. doi:10.1016/j.jpain.2013.08.007

8. Haack M, Mullington JM. Sustained sleep restriction reduces emotional and physical well-being. Pain. 2005;119(1-3):56-64. doi:10.1016/j.pain.2005.09.011

9. Zaccaro A, Piarulli A, Laurino M, et al. How breath-control can change your life: a systematic review on psycho-physiological correlates of slow breathing. Front Hum Neurosci. 2018;12:353. doi:10.3389/fnhum.2018.00353

10. Balban MY, Neri E, Kogon MM, et al. Brief structured respiration practices enhance mood and reduce physiological arousal. Cell Rep Med. 2023;4(1):100895. doi:10.1016/j.xcrm.2022.100895.

11. Liang Z, Ding Z, Wang D, et al. Cryotherapy for rehabilitation after total knee arthroplasty: a comprehensive systematic review and meta-analysis. Orthop Surg. 2024;16(12):2897-2915. doi:10.1111/os.14266

12. Wei G, Shang Z, Li Y, et al. Effects of lower-limb active resistance exercise on mobility, physical function, knee strength and pain intensity in patients with total knee arthroplasty: a systematic review and meta-analysis. BMC Musculoskelet Disord. 2024;25:730. doi:10.1186/s12891-024-07845-9

13. Ickert EC, Griswold D, Ross O, Dudash S, Duchon C, Learman K. Effects of kinesiotaping during early post-operative rehabilitation in individuals who underwent a total knee arthroplasty: a systematic review and meta-analysis of randomized control trials. Clin Rehabil. 2024;38(6):732-748. doi:10.1177/02692155241230894

14. Baas DC, van Aalderen-Wichers JC, van der Goot TH, Verhagen RJ. The effect of pain neuroscience education on chronic postsurgical pain after total knee arthroplasty: a randomized controlled trial. Acta Orthop. 2024;95:485-491. doi:10.2340/17453674.2024.41346

15. National Institute for Health and Care Excellence. Joint replacement (primary): hip, knee and shoulder. NICE guideline NG157. Published June 4, 2020. Last reviewed December 19, 2024. Accessed September 6, 2026. https://www.nice.org.uk/guidance/ng157

16. American Academy of Orthopaedic Surgeons. Activities after total knee replacement. OrthoInfo. Accessed September 6, 2026.

https://www.orthoinfo.org/en/recovery/activities-after-knee-replacement/

17. American Academy of Orthopaedic Surgeons. Total knee replacement exercise guide. OrthoInfo. Accessed September 6, 2026. https://www.orthoinfo.org/recovery/total-knee-replacement-exercise-guide/

Made in the USA
Monee, IL
04 November 2026

67383569R10049